How I Quit Smoking

In 31 Days

After Smoking

For 32 Years

By Michael T. Petro, Jr.

How I Quit Smoking In 31 Days

After Smoking For 32 Years

Copyright © 2012 by Michael T. Petro, Jr.

All rights reserved solely by the author. No part of this book may be reproduced, stored in a retrieval system, or transmitted in any other form or by any means, including electronic, mechanical, photocopy, recording, scanning, or any other, without prior written permission from the author, except for reviewers and researchers who may quote brief passages.

Nothing in this book is to be considered medical advice. The author's simple, natural plan has been personally tested and proven to be safe and effective. However, due to individual variation, the reader is encouraged to share the contents of this book with a physician or other health care professional before implementing this plan.

ISBN-10: 0-9650411-4-X

ISBN-13: 978-0-9650411-4-0

Published by **Petro Publications**

www.PetroPublications.com

Table of Contents

Dear Future Non-Smoker:..5

What To Do Before You Quit!

Step One: Make A Firm Commitment To Quit!...............................6

Step Two: Set A Specific Time & Date To Quit!.............................6

Step Three: Brainwash Yourself!...8

Step Four: Talk To Your Doctor, Dentist & Others!......................11

Step Five: Tell Your Family, Friends & Coworkers!......................12

Step Six: Start Smoking Fewer Cigarettes!..................................13

Step Seven: Don't Smoke In Cars & Bars!...................................14

Step Eight: Carry Gum Or Candy With You!................................16

Step Nine: Talk To Yourself About Specific Facts!......................17

What To Do After You Quit!

Step Ten: Give Yourself A 30-Day Grace Period!...................19

Step Eleven: Take It One Day At A Time!..................20

Step Twelve: Enjoy The Benefits Of A Non-Smoker!...................21

Enjoy The Physical & Mental Benefits!...................21

Enjoy The Financial Benefits!...................24

Dear Future Non-Smoker:

Like many nicotine addicts, I had quit smoking numerous times, only to relapse over and over again. On August 1, 1991, I quit smoking – for the last time! On August 1, 2011, I celebrated 20 years as a non-smoker, and remain serenely smoke-free today.

If I can do it, you can do it. How do I know this? Because I smoked for 32 years, and smoked about two packs each and every day for many, many years. So, it makes no difference how long you have been smoking, and it doesn't make any difference how many cigarettes you smoke each day. If you really want to quit, you can quit. Now let's review the specific steps I took to quit smoking – for good - in just 31 days.

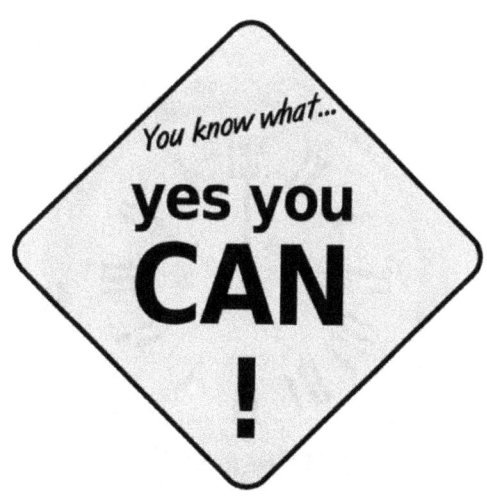

What To Do Before You Quit!

Step One: Make A Firm Commitment to Quit!

You must make a firm, irreversible commitment to quit smoking. I said to myself, "This decision is one of the most important decisions of my life. I'm going to quit smoking, and, once I quit, I'm not going to have another cigarette again - ever - period! Once I quit, I'm not going to smoke another cigarette again no matter how difficult it may become! The physical, emotional, and financial damage caused by smoking is just too high a price to pay!"

Step Two: Set A Specific Time & Date to Quit!

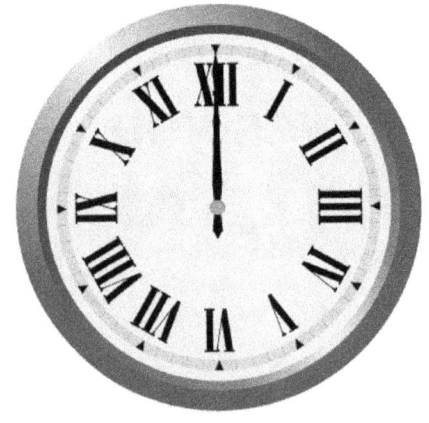

Once the commitment is made - and there is no turning back, you must take the next step and set a specific time and date to quit. I decided to quit at midnight at the end of the 31st day. You may decide to quit in 15 days, or perhaps 45 days. It's up to you. The most important thing to do is set a specific time and date and stick to them. Once the time and date are set, do not change them. You have just made a contract with yourself. So think about it carefully. Choose a time and date you are comfortable with, but choose a date that's not too soon. You must allow yourself ample time for preparation. Also, do not set a date too far into the future, or your motivation to quit may dissipate.

I found 31 days to be best for me, although I played with the idea for about two weeks before I got up enough courage to set a date. So, on July 1, 1991, I set August 1, 1991, as my date to quit. (There are 31 days in the month of July, and I stopped smoking at midnight on the 31st of July, and became smoke-free at 12:00:01 on August 1, 1991) I was literally smoking cigarette butts out of the ashtray up to the very last second.

Step Three: Brainwash Yourself!

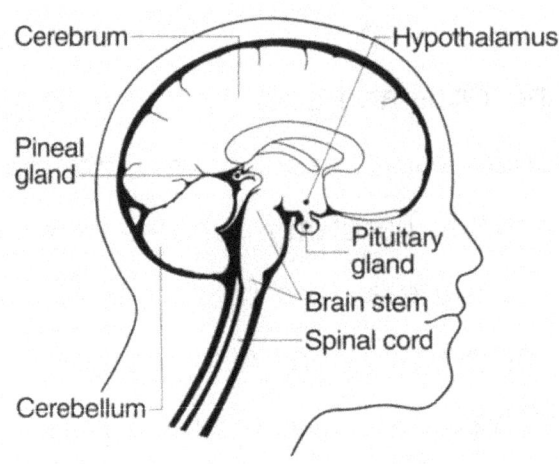

Let's say you picked a 31-day countdown to arrive at your date to quit smoking. Next, make a trip to the library and search out material that explains in detail the health hazards that smokers suffer. For example, read the **Surgeon General's Report on Smoking and Tobacco Use**. Ask the librarian for assistance in finding similar material, including videos or DVDs. Call the Center's For Disease Control and Prevention, or CDC (1-800-232-4636), and ask for a copy of the booklet, **How Tobacco Smoke Causes Disease: What It Means To You**. If you have a computer, go to CDC.gov and review the **Surgeon General's Report on Smoking and Tobacco Use** online. Also, read online the free **Quit Guide** available at SmokeFree.gov.

Read the best material you can get your hands on. That's what I did. Saturate your mind with vivid details that describe the enormous damage you are inflicting upon yourself as you smoke. Continue this "self-brainwashing" procedure to build up psychological momentum as you approach the day you will cease smoking. The more you read, the more you will want to quit – and you must possess a strong commitment as you race toward, and past, your deadline.

Search the World Wide Web with the search words "How to quit smoking." Explore the many educational websites that are available for free! Go to YouTube.com and type in "Tips from former smokers." You will find many 31-second anti-smoking ads. Most heartbreaking are the videos featuring Terrie Hall, who started smoking as a teenager. You will see what Terrie Hall looked like before smoking ravaged her body, and what she looks like today after years of smoking.

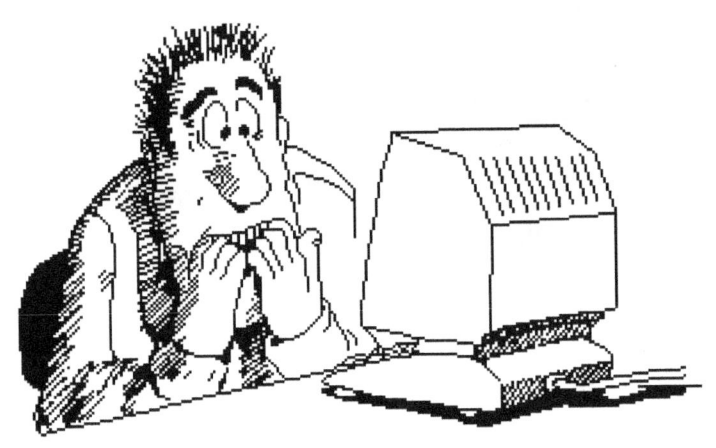

Warning: These videos are not for the fainthearted!

You can view videos of Terrie Hall at the below three web addresses:

http://www.youtube.com/watch?v=PzhNCbbnv5A&feature=relmfu

http://www.youtube.com/watch?v=qNiBZt1hEzA&feature=relmfu

http://www.youtube.com/watch?v=5zWB4dLYChM

If you lack the deep commitment necessary to quit smoking, review these videos at least once each day. Burn the images of this woman into your conscious mind and your subconscious mind. You will never look at cigarette smoking the same again. I guarantee it!

Step Four: Talk To Your Physician, Dentist & Others!

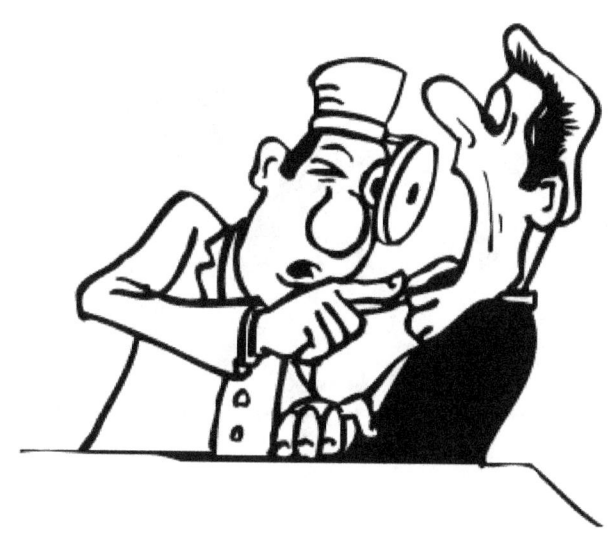

Talk to your physician and dentist and notify them of your plan to quit smoking. They may give you some good advice, some encouragement, and may suggest some good material to read that may help you brainwash yourself into becoming a non-smoker! They may even let you know how your quitting will affect some health conditions you may have. They may also provide information on many serious health conditions you may avoid as a direct result of becoming a non-smoker. Discuss your plans with other health care professionals as well. They may be an excellent source of support, encouragement, and educational material.

Step Five: Tell Everyone About Your Plan To Quit!

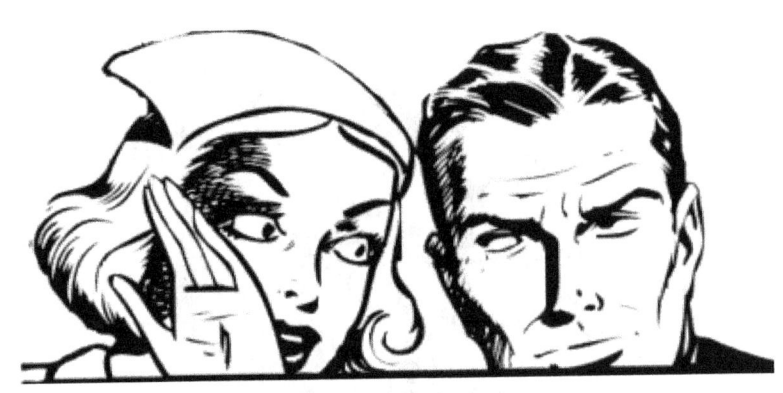

With your commitment firmly made, your time and date set, and your brainwashing procedure in place, tell everyone you know the specific time and date you have set to become a non-smoker. Tell your family, your friends, your neighbors, and your coworkers. This is one of the most effective ways to burn your bridges behind you. When you inform all the important people in your life that you intend to quit, it becomes extremely difficult to backtrack. It simply becomes too embarrassing to smoke again after you have told everyone you know that you have made a firm commitment to quit. You may be surprised at the support and encouragement you will receive. You may even learn that some of the people you talk to are former smokers. They may be an excellent source of support and encouragement, and may even give you a few good tips on how they succeeded in becoming non-smokers.

Step Six: Start Smoking Fewer Cigarettes!

Reduce the number of cigarettes you smoke the first week. I went from smoking two packs each day to one and one-half packs during the first week of my 31-day countdown. The second week I dropped to about one pack each day. This was maintained during the third week as well, and during the fourth and last week I dropped down to about one-half pack per day. This weaning process will help both your body and your mind adjust to a decreasing intake of nicotine. It will help prepare you for the day when you will have no nicotine coming into your system.

Step Seven: Don't Smoke In Cars & Bars!

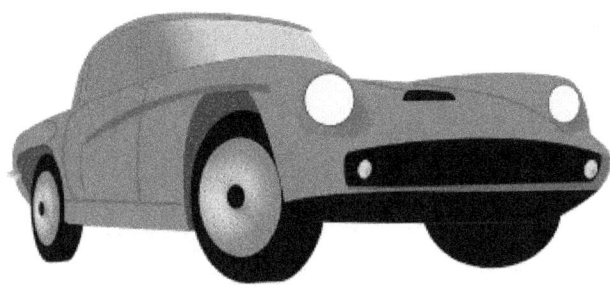

Most people who smoke and drive will smoke in their vehicles as they drive to and from work, and as they drive to and from other locations. If this is true for you, and you have set, for example, a 31-day countdown, perhaps by day seven you should stop carrying cigarettes in your car, truck, van, or other vehicle.

I spent about two hours each day in my vehicle driving round-trip to and from work. So, when the weaning process began, I spent about one hour smoke-free driving to work each morning, and another hour smoke-free driving home in the late afternoon. By declaring my car a smoke-free vehicle during the first week of my countdown, I became accustomed to the idea of not smoking for at least one hour or so – at least twice each day. Although I did not go to bars and nightclubs at the time I began weaning myself from tobacco, I would often dine at a local restaurant. At this particular restaurant I would usually sit at the counter, eat a meal, and chat with the usual crowd that came up there each evening.

In addition to notifying these friends and acquaintances of my intent to quit smoking, I actually stopped smoking at that restaurant about two weeks before reaching my non-smoking deadline. This was an excellent opportunity to wean myself. When I began weaning myself back in July, 1991, smoking was still permitted in most public places. Times have certainly changed. However, if you frequent public or private places that allow smoking, at some point in your countdown - perhaps midway or sooner - stop smoking at these locations. This constitutes excellent practice in preparing yourself to become a non-smoker.

Step Eight: Carry Gum Or Candy With You!

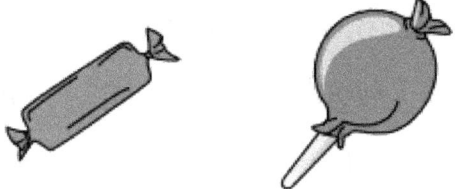

You may need to check with your doctor and dentist about this. If your doctor and dentist say it is OK for you to carry gum or candy with you temporarily during - and perhaps shortly after - your weaning process, begin doing so the first day of your countdown. When you begin weaning yourself and the urge for a cigarette comes upon you, instead of reaching for a cigarette, you can reach for a stick of gum or a piece of candy - such as a lollipop! The advantage of the lollipop is that you can handle it nearly the same way you handle a cigarette.

If you are concerned about adding sweets to your diet, you may want to buy some non-sugar snacks at your local health food store. They could serve as a good supplement to, or perhaps a good substitute for, gum and candy. You could also purchase sugarless gum, as well as fresh fruit!

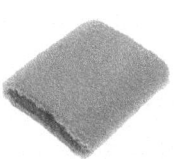 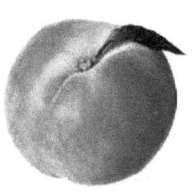 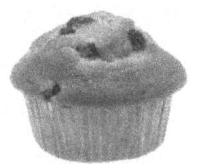

Step Nine: Talk To Yourself About Specific Facts!

As you get closer to day 31 in your 31-day countdown to a smoke-free life, your anxiety level may begin to build. This will be a good time to rehearse some of the specific facts you learned during your self-brain-washing process. Recalling some specific facts will come in handy during moments of weakness.

For example, I reminded myself that most of the anxiety will be greatly reduced after just the first three days as a non-smoker. It is during this three-day period that your body will detoxify itself from most - if not all - of the residual nicotine. So, this is when the strongest withdrawals will be felt. To rid myself of cigarettes and protect my health, I decided that I could handle most any kind of withdrawal symptoms for only three days.

Secondly, I frequently reminded myself that the greatest intensity of withdrawals lasts only for a few seconds. So, I would only need to search for a stick of gum, or for a piece of candy. By the time I would locate and place the gum or candy into my mouth, the craving will have already begun to subside. If no gum or candy was available, I would only need to breathe deeply and slowly and tell myself to hang on for just a few seconds. I decided I could stand on my head for a few seconds, if that is what was necessary to rid myself of this health-destroying addiction.

Thirdly, I often reminded myself that many psychologists believe it takes only about 21 days, or three weeks, to reprogram your subconscious mind. So, by brainwashing myself for 31 days, or more than four weeks, I had actually reprogrammed myself to be a non-smoker BEFORE I actually quit smoking. I recreated my self-image from that of a smoker to that of a non-smoker while slowly decreasing my nicotine intake.

This new self-image comes in handy when someone asks you for a light or for a cigarette after you quit. You simply respond by saying what any non-smoker would say: **"Sorry, I don't smoke!"** Just hearing yourself saying those words will be a huge boast to your self-image. During your first day without cigarettes, you will truly be a non-smoker. You will truly be a new person. Engaging in such self-talk before you actually quit constitutes good practice that will really pay off when you find yourself craving a cigarette soon after you become a non-smoker.

What To Do After You Quit!

Step Ten: Give Yourself A 30-Day Grace Period!

During my first 30 days as a non-smoker, I allowed myself (within reason) to consume a lot of candy, gum, and other snacks. Again, you need to check with your doctor and dentist before you do this. I had other snacks on hand as well, such as popcorn, potato chips, and health food bars. For the first 30 days as a non-smoker, I always had a good supply of these goodies in my pocket, my car, my desk at work, and in my cupboard at home. If you don't want to eat the junk food that I ate, check with your doctor, dentist, and the knowledgeable sales people you usually find at a health food store. You may find a delightful variety of healthy and delicious alternatives!

In addition, you will find great wisdom in the 12-Step Program of Alcoholics Anonymous (AA). Reading AA literature during your first 30 days, and perhaps thereafter, can be very helpful in overcoming most any addiction! You can also check out Nicotine-Anonymous.org.

Step Eleven: Take It One Day At A Time!

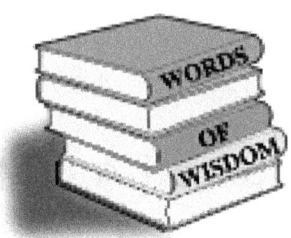

You may not have thought about your cigarette habit in these terms, but your battle with nicotine is not much different from the battles others have fought and won against other addictive substances. This includes highly addictive substances such as alcohol, cocaine, and heroin. So, when you quit smoking, you will not only be a non-smoker, you will be a recovering nicotine addict! For this reason you may find the wisdom of the AA 12-Step Program very beneficial.

The helpful hint that I found most useful from AA was the adage, **"Take It One Day At A Time!"** This adage keeps you from being overwhelmed in the event you see yourself as a struggling non-smoker for an extended period of time. In moments of weakness you can easily tell yourself, ***"No matter what happens, TODAY I will be smoke-free!"*** Concern yourself with being a non-smoker just for today. Tomorrow will take care of itself!

Step Twelve: Enjoy The Benefits Of A Non-Smoker!

Enjoy The Physical And Mental Benefits!

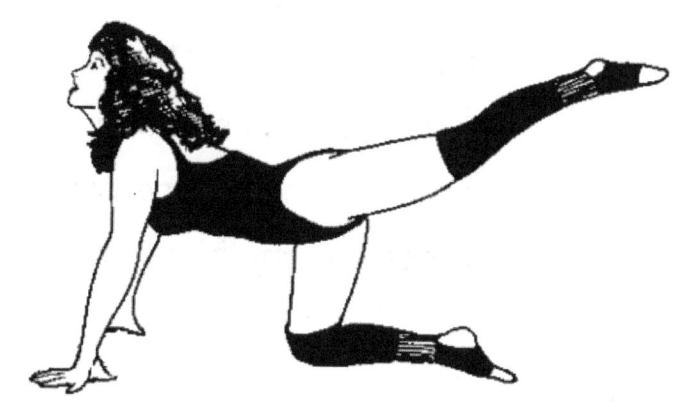

About 10 days after I quit smoking, I discovered that I had lost my smoker's cough. That was simply amazing! I had that smoker's cough for more years than I could remember, perhaps more than a decade. It was great to wake up in the morning and not hack my lungs out. I really couldn't believe that I had lost that killer cough in such a short period of time. The loss of my smoker's cough was the first health benefit I had noticed. But a second immediate benefit was pointed out to me by a coworker. About the same time that I had stopped coughing in the morning, a coworker made a startling observation. As I walked into his office to talk to him, my coworker, who was a fairly dark-skinned man of Middle-Eastern descent, said, *"Your skin has a pinkish tint to it. You don't look as white as you did before."*

Wow! That was great news! I knew exactly what that meant, and I shared it with him. I said, in straightforward terms, *"That's a sign that I'm now getting more oxygen to my skin. When I was smoking, my blood was filled with the many poisonous gases found in burning tobacco and cigarette paper. Without those poisonous gases in my blood, there's more room for nourishing oxygen."*

It really is true. When you quit smoking, in just a short time you begin to experience some amazing changes in yourself. Others will begin to notice them, too. When there's more oxygen in your blood, there's more oxygen being delivered to every cell in your body, including your skin. You will be getting more oxygen into your lungs, heart, brain, liver, and every other organ in your body. With this increase in life-giving oxygen you become more resistant to many aliments, including viral and bacterial infections. Also, when you do get sick or injured, the increased oxygen level will accelerate the healing process. Ask your doctor if all this is really true!

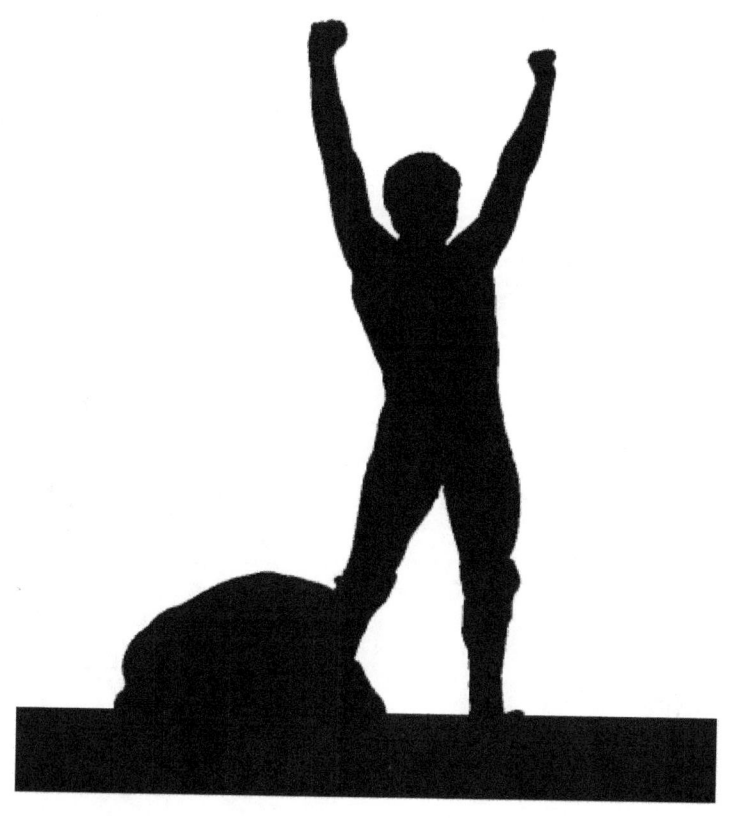

ENJOY THE NEW YOU!

There's no question about it! As a non-smoker, in less than two short weeks, you can look healthier, you can feel healthier, and you can actually be healthier. Rejoice in your new found self with your family, your friends, your neighbors, and your coworkers.

Enjoy The Financial Benefits!

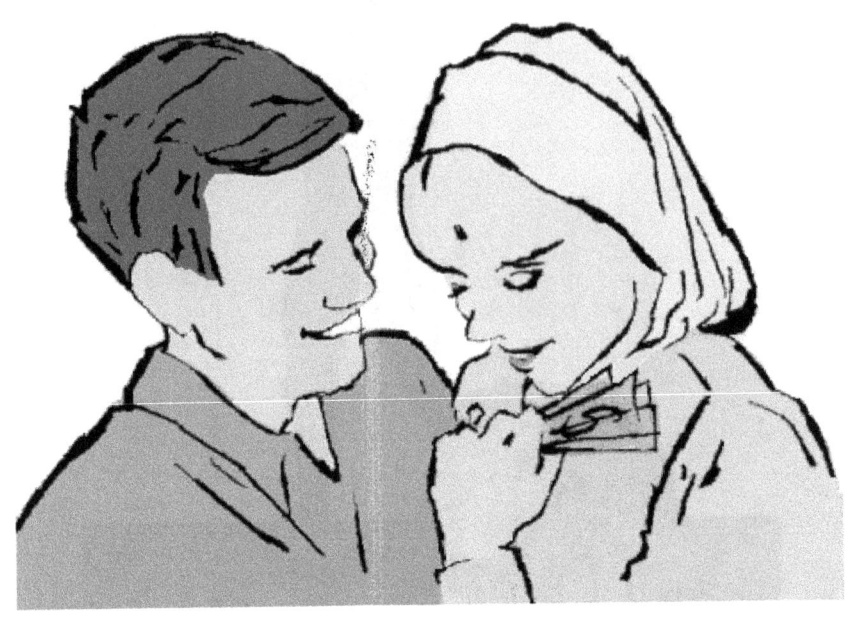

When I quit smoking in 1991, the average cost of a pack of cigarettes was about $2.00. By not smoking two packs per day from 1991 to 2011, I saved $4.00 per day, $120.00 per month, about $1,450.00 per year, and about $29,000.00 over a 20-year period – if the price had remained at only $2.00 per pack. However, today, in 2012, the average cost of a pack of cigarettes in the USA is about $5.00 per pack. If you smoke two packs per day, as a non-smoker you will save $10.00 per day, $300.00 per month, and about $3,600.00 per year! WOW! What will you do with all that extra money? Make your plans to quit NOW!

www.ingramcontent.com/pod-product-compliance
Lightning Source LLC
Chambersburg PA
CBHW081026040426
42444CB00014B/3369